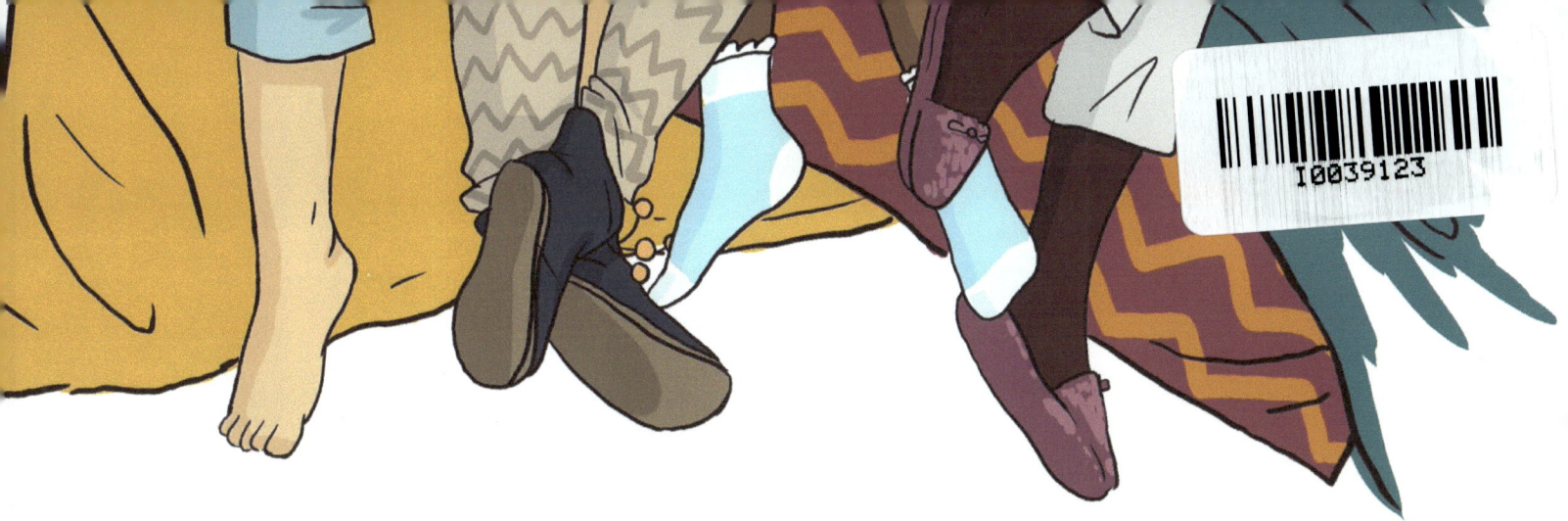

THE Book OF Cuddles

WRITTEN BY Dr. Yoni Alkan

ILLUSTRATED BY Cecilia Li

with foreword by MADELON GUINAZZO and MARCIA BACZYNSKI

CONTENTS

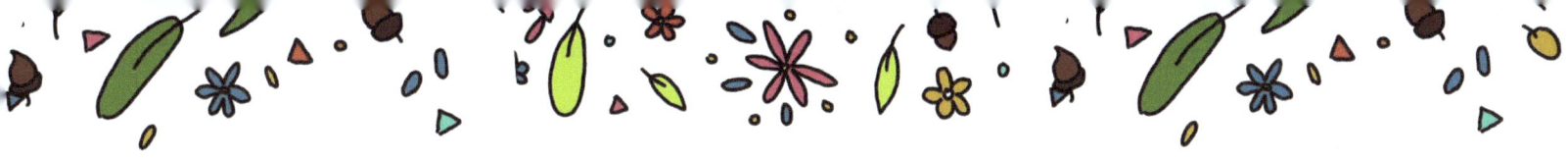

Preface   v

Introduction : What is Cuddling?   vii

Foreword: Let's Talk About Consent   xi

How to Experience Better Touch   1

Touching with Intent   2

Touch is Bi-Directional   3

Try Out Different Kinds of Touch   3

CUDDLING POSITIONS

One-on-One Positions   5

Buddies   6

Back to Back   8

Face Time   10

Storytime   12

Spooning   14

Gonna Be Okay   16

Recumbent Bicycle   18

Listen to the beat   20

Safe Cradle   22

Lying Down Safe Cradle   24

Sleeping Kid   26

Mirror Image   28

Hugs   31

Seatbelt Hug   32

Envelope Hug   34

Blanket Hug   36

Group Cuddles   39

Hand Loop   40

Massage Train   42

Spoon Drawer   44

Laugh Circle   46

Puppy Pile   48

Cuddle-cule   50

Epilogue   52

Acknowledgements   53

PREFACE

Welcome to the Book of Cuddles!

This book is an instructional book about cuddling. It's devised to help people feel more comfortable sharing touch with one another. We invite you to look through the book, find positions that interest you, and try them out with willing friends.

Today, more than ever, we need more safe, caring, compassionate touch. Many people lack touch—and they might not even know it. I know this might sound like hippie talk, but it's incredible how touch can affect our bodies and spirits. People seek cuddles for various reasons: they want companionship, attention, a safe space to receive positive touch, or just fun. Cuddling can provide those—and cuddling can change people's lives.

The first part of the book discusses cuddling, consent, and touch in ways that will allow you to enhance your cuddling game and bring safer and better touch into your life.

The second part has a variety of positions you can try out, along with directions for how and where (such as on a couch or mattress). Each position also includes some pro tips for approaching each position and finding what's best and most comfortable for you.

Every position is also sorted by level of intimacy. These levels change from person to person, depending how you cuddle, but they are there as a guideline. The further you go into the book, the more intimate the positions get.

The Book of Cuddles is intended for all people, regardless of gender, age, body type, or ability. Some positions might work for you and others might not. Try things out, be curious, and find what is good for you.

Big hugs (if you'd like some),
Yoni and Cecilia

INTRODUCTION: WHAT IS CUDDLING?

By Madelon Guinazzo

Cuddling is what many humans do instinctively as children. The human psyche needs to feel secure to grow strong—physically, mentally, and emotionally. We also cuddle naturally as parents, friends, grandparents, and lovers. It is what people in bodies do when they enjoy being close with other people in bodies. People cuddle when they are happy, sad, or scared; it lets us express joy or makes us feel better. Cuddling is playful, sweet, silly, and soothing. In fact, when people feel safe and cared for enough to cuddle, they usually begin to open up and let out some of the weight they've been carrying inside. Cuddling is both uniquely individual and universal, ancient and new, primal and progressive.

Physiologically, cuddling soothes the nervous system and calms the amygdala (which is responsible for some emotions and survival instincts). It activates the parasympathetic response, which controls things like heart rate and intestinal activity. It produces oxytocin and vasopressin, which counteract cortisol and adrenaline (so-called stress hormones). It takes us out of the "fight, flight, or freeze response" and into feelings of well-being, trust and confidence. It brings balance and perspective. The relaxation of cuddling can be like a spring thaw that brings new life and vitality. If you're doing it well, it's hard to take yourself too seriously or put pressure on yourself when cuddling. It is the readily available, low-cost, low side-effect antidote to the rat race, with its urgent calls to do everything "bigger, better, faster, harder, more!" Cuddling whispers to us, "All is well. You have everything you need, right now, in this moment."

What scientists and cuddlers alike are discovering is that children's need for cuddling is something that we never outgrow. Cuddling isn't just for children—or just for lovers, either. We greatly limit our access to this basic, essential human nutrient if we insist on only doing it within a sexual relationship. Cuddling has the potential to expand our definition of intimacy. And, like sex, consent is cuddling's best buddy. We might not have had to think about that part as kids, but as adults we must own our rights and responsibilities about our choices. When two sovereign rulers of two bodies come together with the alliance of consent, they each become the most benevolent versions of themselves and create a healthy place for their inner children to play.

So what is cuddling? It is the language of the body, heart, mind, and soul. When you're a bit down, it is the friend who comes over with homemade soup and a fun movie, says "Tell me all about it," and doesn't try to fix you. Consensual cuddling helps us see the best in others. It leads to pillow talk: the things we say to people when we trust them. It is an invitation to be who we are without reservation. It's not the key to happiness or world peace. It is an abundant resource that soothes us and smooths the rough edges of life. It gives us practice in communicating better and being kinder to ourselves and others. It is a state of mind and a way of being. Cuddling is the thing for which there are no words—and for which no words are needed.

Thank you, Cecilia and Yoni, for this beautiful book. Use this book to explore your options and to enjoy your life, dear reader.

Madelon Guinazzo is the co-founder of Cuddlist and the creator of certification training

www.cuddlist.com

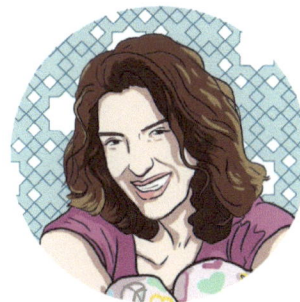

X

FOREWORD: LET'S TALK ABOUT CONSENT

By Marcia Baczynski

Consent is the backbone of a delightful cuddle experience. Knowing that everyone wants to be there, doing what they are doing, allows each person to relax more fully into the experience, without worrying if they are taking up too much space, or doing something unwelcome.

Contrary to popular belief, consent doesn't have to be a heavy topic or involve endless conversations. It is simply an agreement about how we're going to play or share space together.

Kids seem to be really good at creating agreements:

> "Let's play tag! You be it!"
> "No, I don't wanna be it!"
> "Okay, I'll be it!"

And they're off!

This is an example of a game where the rules are understood. But if you watch kids, they build elaborate worlds with rules and desires that change constantly and are inscrutable to outsiders. They improvise and they throw stuff out there and they keep talking. They fight and sort it out and keep going till they're done or bored or it's time for dinner.
This is consent in action. It's ongoing. You can opt in or out at any time. You might not totally know what you're getting into, but you're building things as you go and checking in with one another. Everyone is being self-ish and generous at the same time, in service of keeping the play going.

There are six key consent skills at play here:

- Saying what you want
- Saying *yes*
- Saying *no*
- Changing your mind
- Listening to the other person as they do the same
- Incorporating ideas and proposing things as the game evolves

When you play, you are inviting the other person in, sharing your enthusiasm for them and the ideas you both have for play. You're giving room to say *yes* or *no* and allowing everyone a voice about what's on the table. And that makes it more fun.

Here are some tips for building cuddly agreements:

• **Try building a rulebook together.** You can use pre-written rules as guidelines (such as the Cuddle Party Rules at http://cuddleparty.com/rules) or make up your own.

• **Ask for what you want.** It's important to put out some ideas about what each of you wants in order to have the most positive experience possible. It can be tempting to go with the first idea ("Wanna spoon?"), but maybe someone wants to be held, or maybe they want to be more active by giving a partial massage while cuddling. Ask for what you *want*, not what you think you can get. Encourage your cuddle buddies to do the same.

• **Stay comfortable.** A good practice for creating consent is to set the agreements within the comfort zone of the least comfortable person. For example, if one person is okay with shirts-off cuddling and another is not, keep your shirts on. If you're spooning and one person is uncomfortable with someone's crotch being near them, they can be the big spoon, or together you can explore other positions that feel good to them.

- **Changing your mind is okay!** Anyone can choose to be done with cuddling at any time, for any reason. Anyone can change their mind about what they want to do at any time, for any reason. That means your cuddle partners might be done before you or need to shift positions, and that's okay.

- **When you are being present to your experience, change is normal.** By saying yes to something, you are not signing a contract saying you'll do it forever or until the other person is done. You're saying "yes for now." When you say no to something, you don't need to close the door on it forever. It can be a "no for now."

- **A *maybe* is a *no*.** Assume that silence, hesitations, dispassionate responses and outright *maybes* mean *no*, at least for now.

With these tips, you can create cuddles that feel good to everyone involved, whether it's two of you or twenty of you.

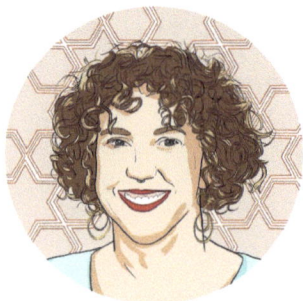

Marcia Baczynski is a sexual communication coach and the co-founder of Cuddle Party

www.askingforwhatyouwant.com

HOW TO EXPERIENCE BETTER TOUCH

Western culture has a complicated relationship with touch. Traditionally, our society does not allow men to explore kind and affectionate touch or nonsexual touch, while most women and nonbinary people have difficulty finding spaces where it is safe for them to experience positive touch and might even find themselves in danger. Additionally, there are marginalized groups that have a hard time finding touch at all because of cultural bias and discrimination around gender, age, body type, race, disability, and other factors.

For some of us, touch is a fundamental part of our lives; for others, it might be a mystery, rarely received or sought out. Some people know instinctively how to touch others, and some have a hard time understanding why others don't enjoy their touch as much or why anyone would want their touch to begin with.

Touch is a basic human need. It is imperative to our well-being and growth. It also allows us to create and maintain connections and relationships with our fellow humans. This section is intended for people who want to better their touch abilities and repertoire so that they and others can enjoy their touch.

TOUCHING WITH INTENT

Just placing your hand on someone else does not constitute "intentional touch." We want to put intention into the way that we touch another person, not just rub our skin against theirs. There are two things to think about when you are practicing intentional touch:

What kind of touch am I giving?
Am I being intentional about it?

First, decide what kind of touch are you going to provide. Will it be a friendly, pleasurable touch? A nurturing touch? A supporting touch? A lover's touch? Your touch can convey a multitude of feelings and messages.

Once you've decided, it's time to convey that message. Concentrate on your fingertips as they move on the other person's body and try to find ways to convey the specific touch you want to share. You can also talk with your touch partner to see if they received the message you intended.

TOUCH IS BI-DIRECTIONAL
Whenever you touch someone, they are also touching you. When you caress someone's forearm with your fingers, their forearm is also caressing your fingers. Keeping that in mind will allow you to focus, so that you too can experience the touch.

TRY OUT DIFFERENT KINDS OF TOUCH
There are countless of ways to exchange touch. Exploring them all can be a great adventure. Which body parts are you touching, and with what kind of touch?

Many of us are used to having our fingers touch someone else's body (for example, their shoulder). But how about the inside of your wrist touching the back of someone's upper arm? Or your cheek against someone's neck? There are endless combinations!

Once you've decided which body part will touch what, you can decide what kind of touch to use. Here are a few ideas:

- Light, gossamer touch
- Strong pressure
- Scratches
- Massage
- Squeezes
- Stationary touch
- Any type of rubs, caresses, strokes, etc.

Combining these two elements through endless trial and error will allow you to discover what makes you feel good.

ONE-ON-ONE
POSITIONS

BUDDIES

INTIMACY
LEVEL

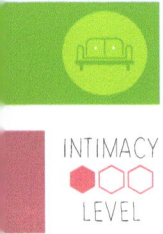

Two people are sitting on the couch, one next to the other, facing forward. Depending on the desired level of closeness, you can sit with no contact, with just the sides of your arms touching, shoulder to shoulder, or holding hands.

This position is a good place to start. You can slowly find your comfort level and see where you want to take it from there.

Pro-Tips

- It's surprising, but hand-holding or playing with each other's hands is actually very intimate. We have many nerve endings in our hands.

- Not having to look at one another allows for a different conversational dynamic.

- One option for moving forward from this position is for one partner to put their head on the other's shoulder.

- It is easy to transfer from this position to other couch-based positions: one of you is already sitting, and the other just needs to shift.

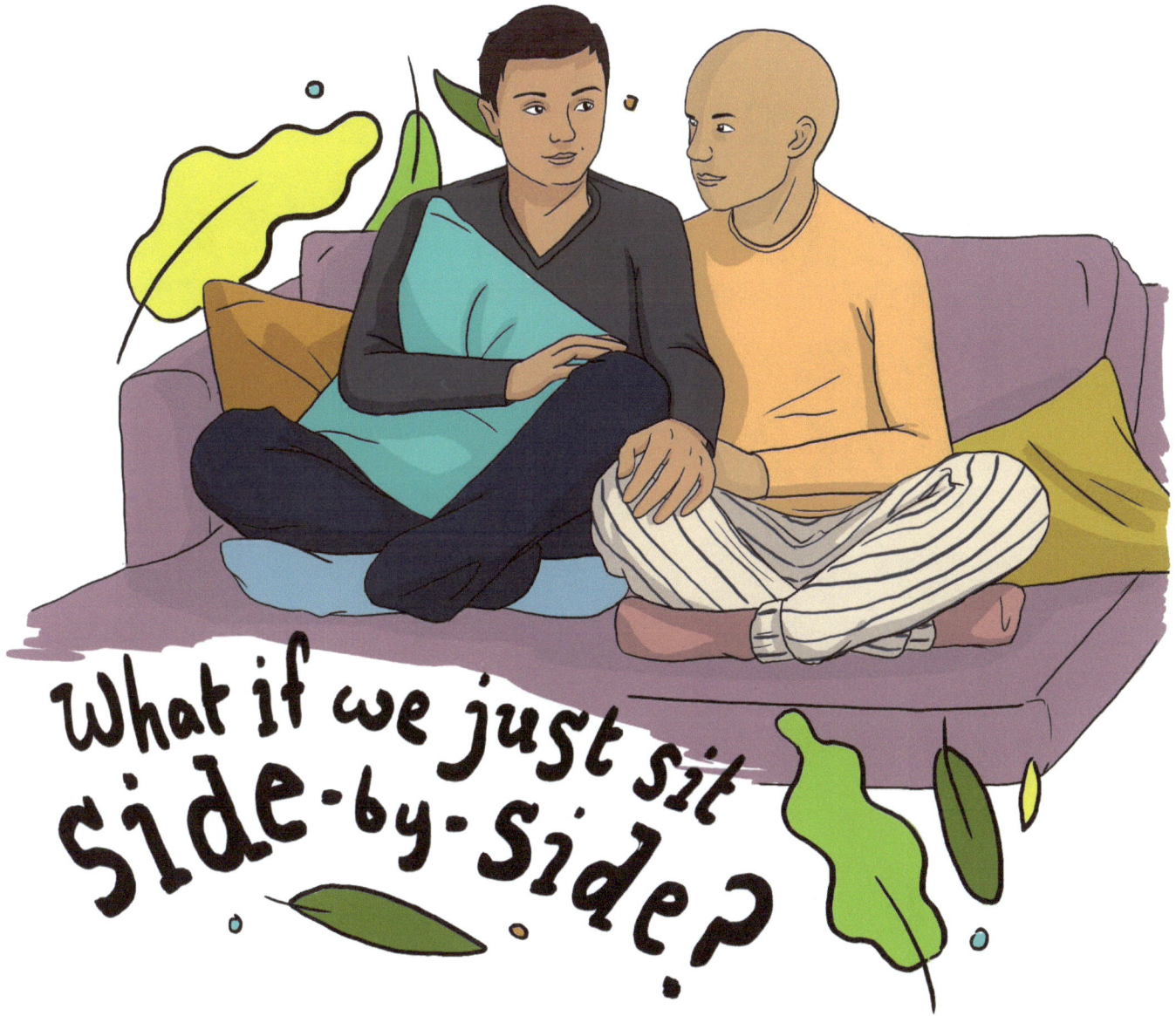

What if we just sit side-by-side?

BACK -to- BACK

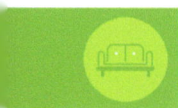

INTIMACY
LEVEL

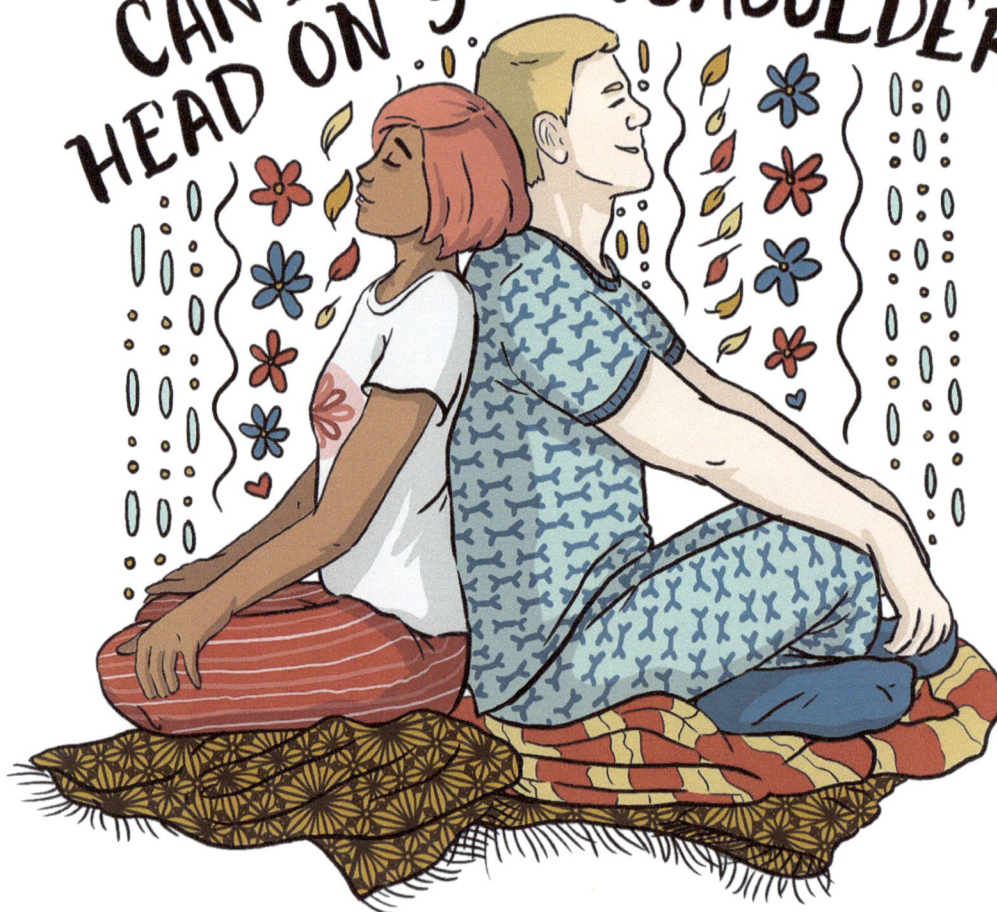

This is another simple position to start building comfort and trust. Both people are sitting upright, facing away from each other and positioned so that your backs are leaning comfortably against one another. This creates touch and pressure between you, without looking at each other. You can also rest the backs of yours heads, one against the other.

Pro-Tips

- Try rocking back and forth in sync, or from side to side, and see how that feels.
- If one person is shorter than the other, they can consider resting their head on the other's shoulder.
- Try breathing together. Synchronize your breath, either together or alternating (one inhales while the other exhales).
- This position is great in silence or to facilitate a conversation.

FACE TIME

INTIMACY
●○○
LEVEL

Sit down cross-legged, possibly with a backrest. Your partner lies down in front of you and rests their head on the spot where your legs cross. This allows you to touch their head, hair, and face. With their comfort and permission, you may also rub their shoulders and/or upper chest.

Pro-Tips

- Put a thin pillow underneath your partner's neck or head for comfort.

- Touching someone's face is a very intimate and private activity. Make sure everyone is comfortable with it and check in to see if it feels good.

- Placing comforting hands on the upper chest and applying slight pressure that corresponds with each exhale might feel good.

- Your partner may bring their arms up to caress your knees or legs.

- Eye gazing could also be interesting, since you are facing in different directions.

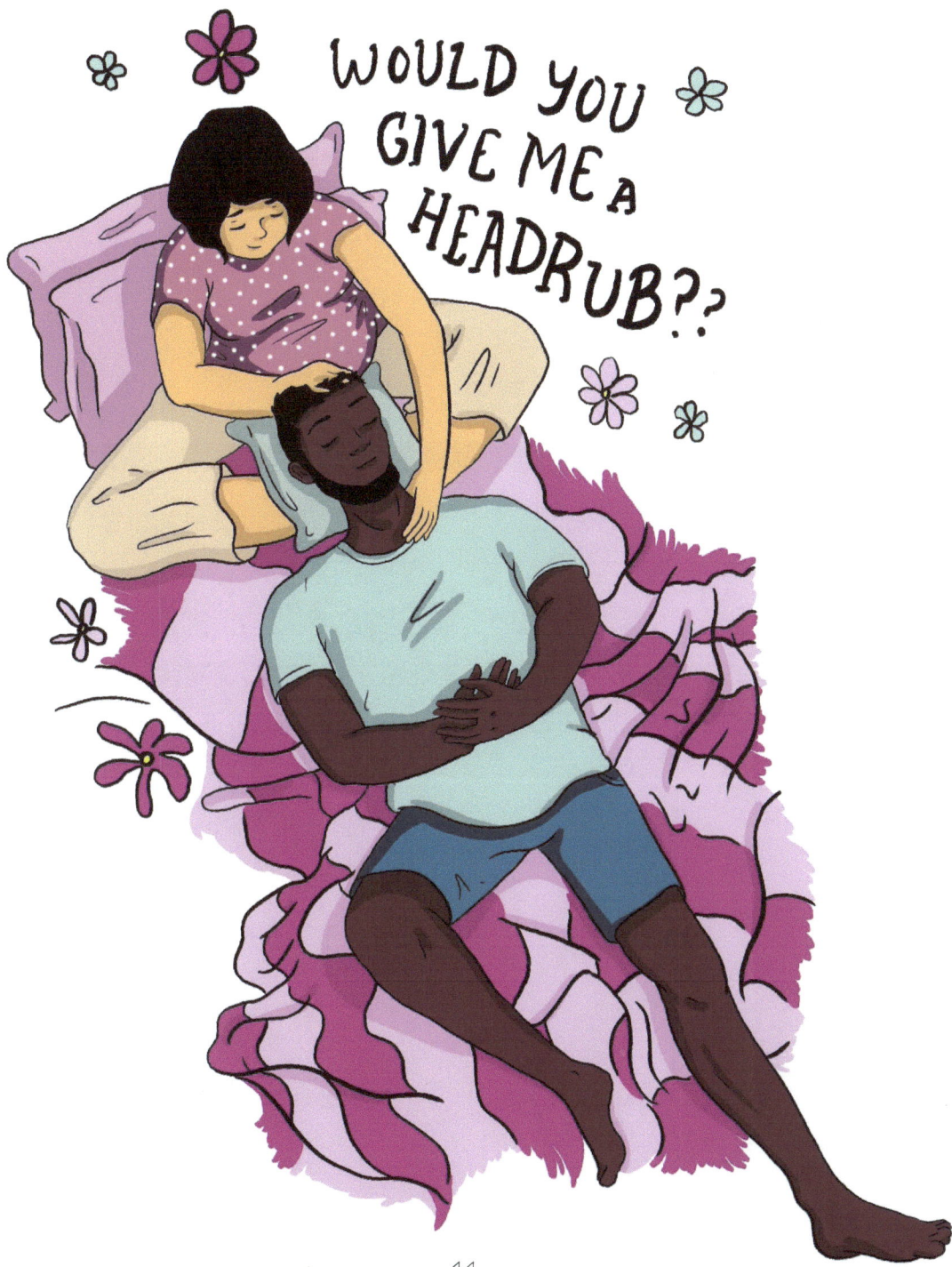

WOULD YOU GIVE ME A HEADRUB??

STORYTIME

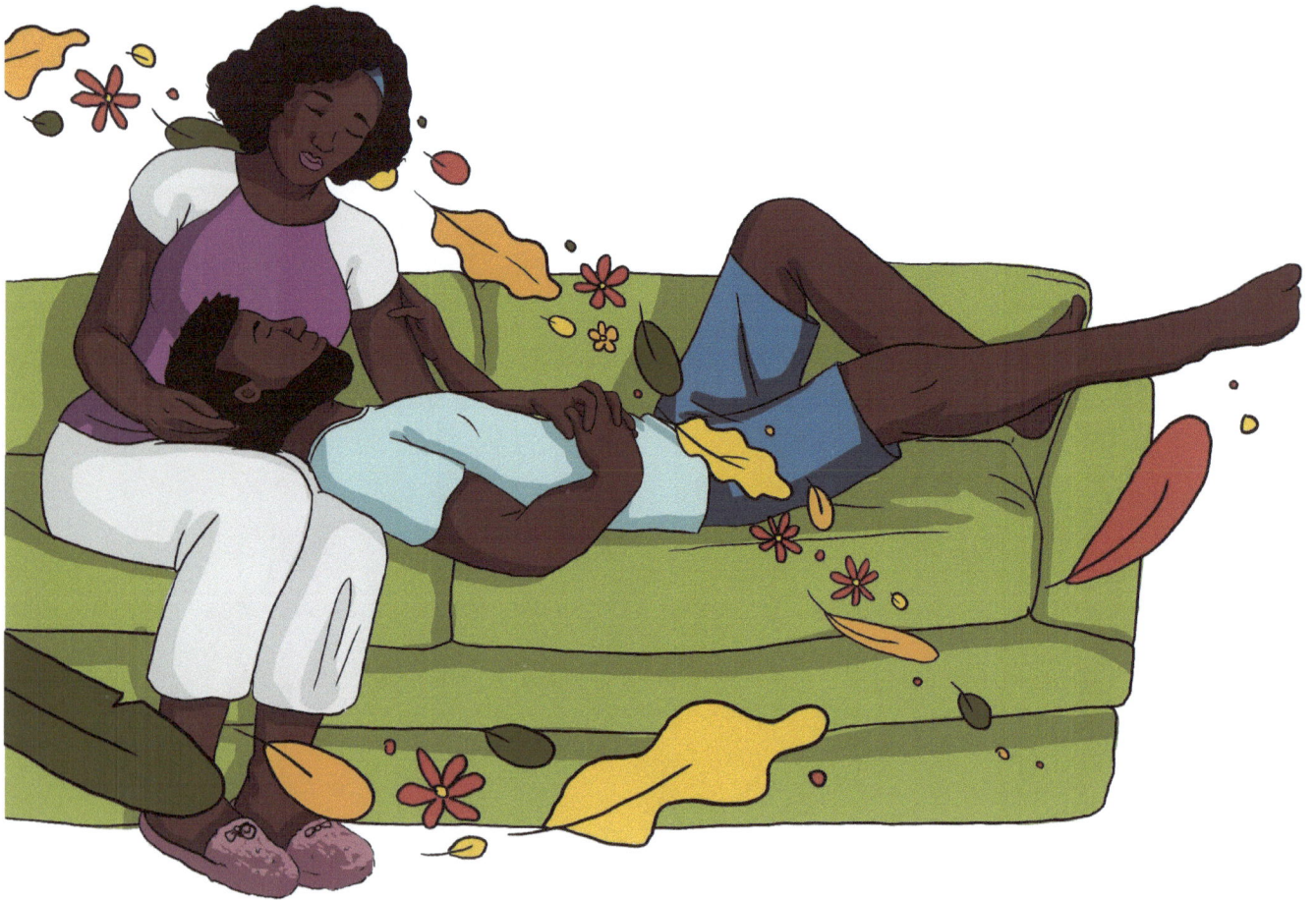

Sit on the couch with your feet on the ground, while your partner lies down and places their head on your lap. Your partner may lie on their back facing up or on one side, depending on their comfort level. This position allows for a comfortable conversation or quiet time.

Pro-Tips

- The person lying down can try this position with their eyes closed or open.

- Playing with someone's face is extremely personal—ask first.

- The intimacy of this position increases greatly if your partner lies with their face sideways toward your body. Make sure both of you are comfortable.

- This is a great position for giving attention to someone. You can make your partner feel very cared for by playing with their hair, shoulders, or arms.

SPOONING

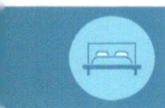

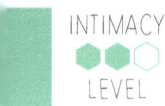

Spooning is one of the most popular cuddling positions. It involves both of you lying on your sides and facing the same direction, with as much body contact as is possible and comfortable. You lie snugly together like two spoons in a drawer. The person behind is called the "Big Spoon," while the person in front is dubbed the "Little Spoon."

Pro-Tips

- To solve the "extra arm" problem, try having the Big Spoon put their bottom arm under the Little Spoon's neck.

- A person's size does not determine whether they should be the Little or the Big Spoon. Try both.

- To avoid arousal, it's possible to place a pillow or a folded blanket between your pelvises.

- The Little Spoon can say where would they like the Big Spoon's top arm to be placed.

- It could be fun to have all four of your feet connected and touching.

- The Little Spoon's stomach and upper chest are a sensitive area—it could feel good to have the Big Spoon's arms or hands on them, if desired.

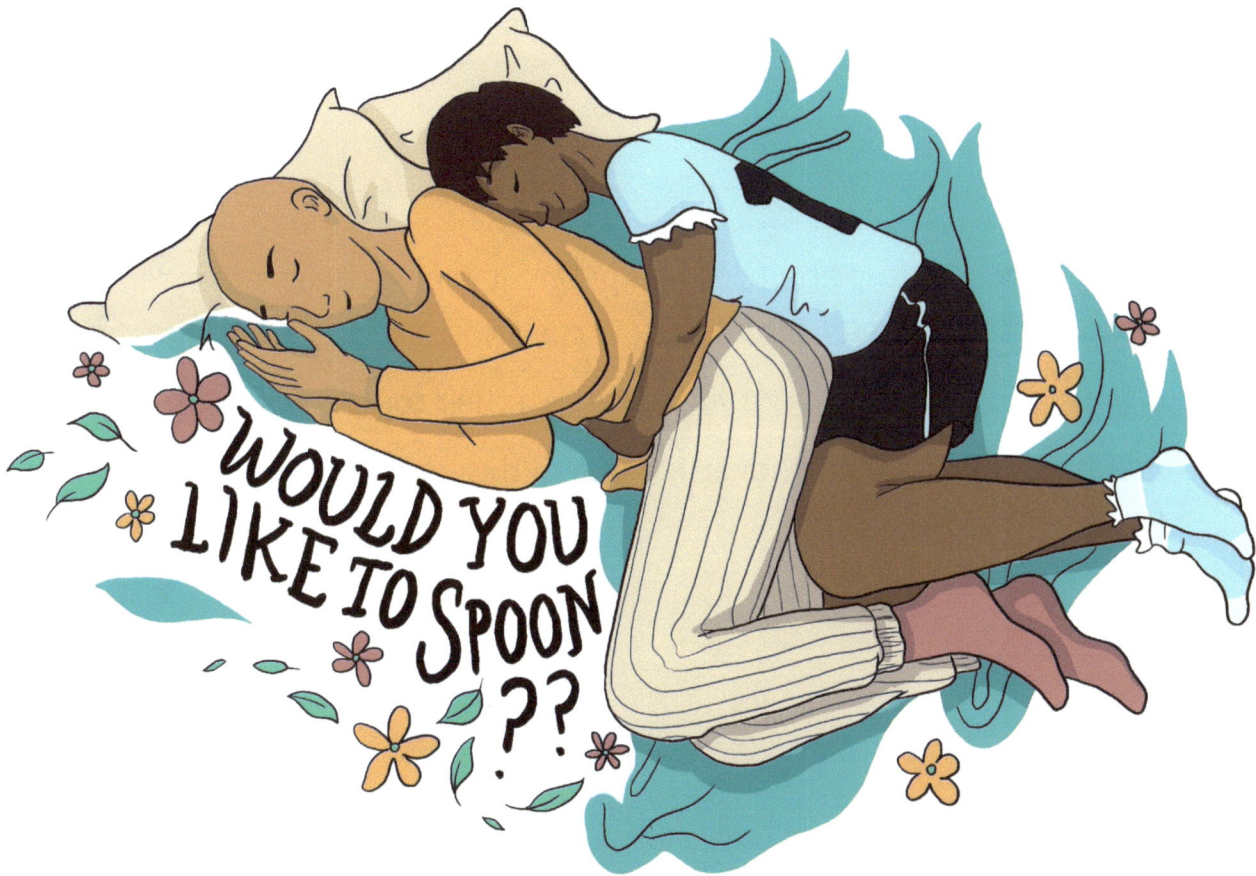

WOULD YOU LIKE TO SPOON??

GONNA BE OKAY

This is a comforting and safe position. Lie on your back. Your partner lies next to you on their side, resting their head on your upper chest. You can place your arm around their back, shoulder, or head, while your other arm is free to rest or hold them in a safe embrace.

Pro-Tips

- Your partner's bottom arm has two options: it can be squeezed underneath their body or placed in front of their body. It can also be stretched behind their back.

- Let your partner know where you would like their top arm to be placed.

- A good way to create additional intimacy in this position is for your partner to place their leg over yours.

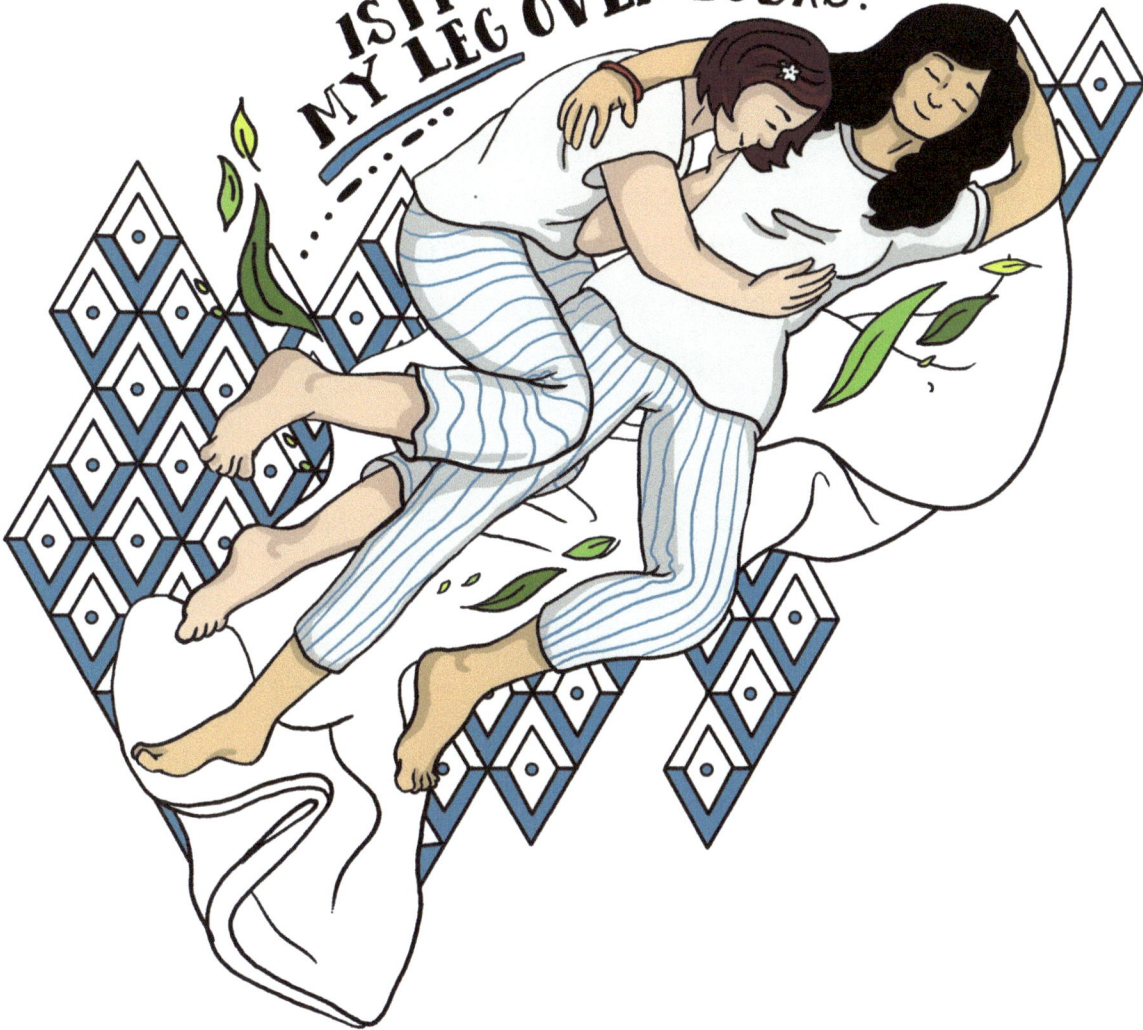

RECUMBENT BICYCLE

Lie down on your stomach with your legs bent, so that the soles of your feet are facing up. Your partner then sits on your bottom, in order to lie down on top of you, facing up, back to back. Now your partner can place their feet on yours so that your soles are touching.

This position allows you to feel the weight of another person on top of you. You can shift where that weight is focused by pushing against one another's feet, or by the top person raising their abdomen or torso slightly.

Pro-Tips

- The top person can try rolling their back over the bottom's back to feel the shift of weight.

- You can try this position with legs closed together or spread apart.

- Many people enjoy feeling another's weight. This position allows you to try it out in a less intimate way.

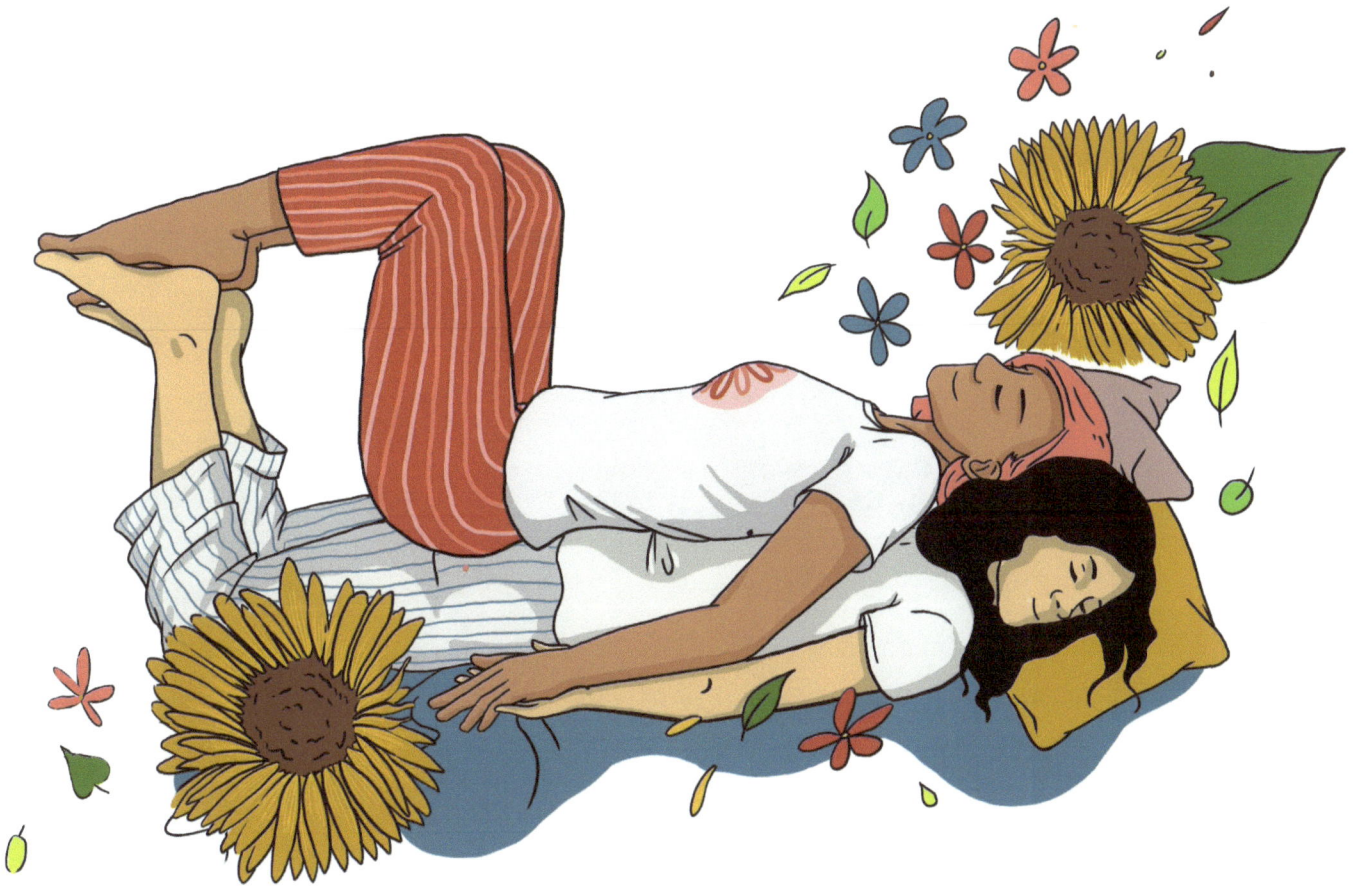

LISTEN TO THE BEAT

INTIMACY
LEVEL

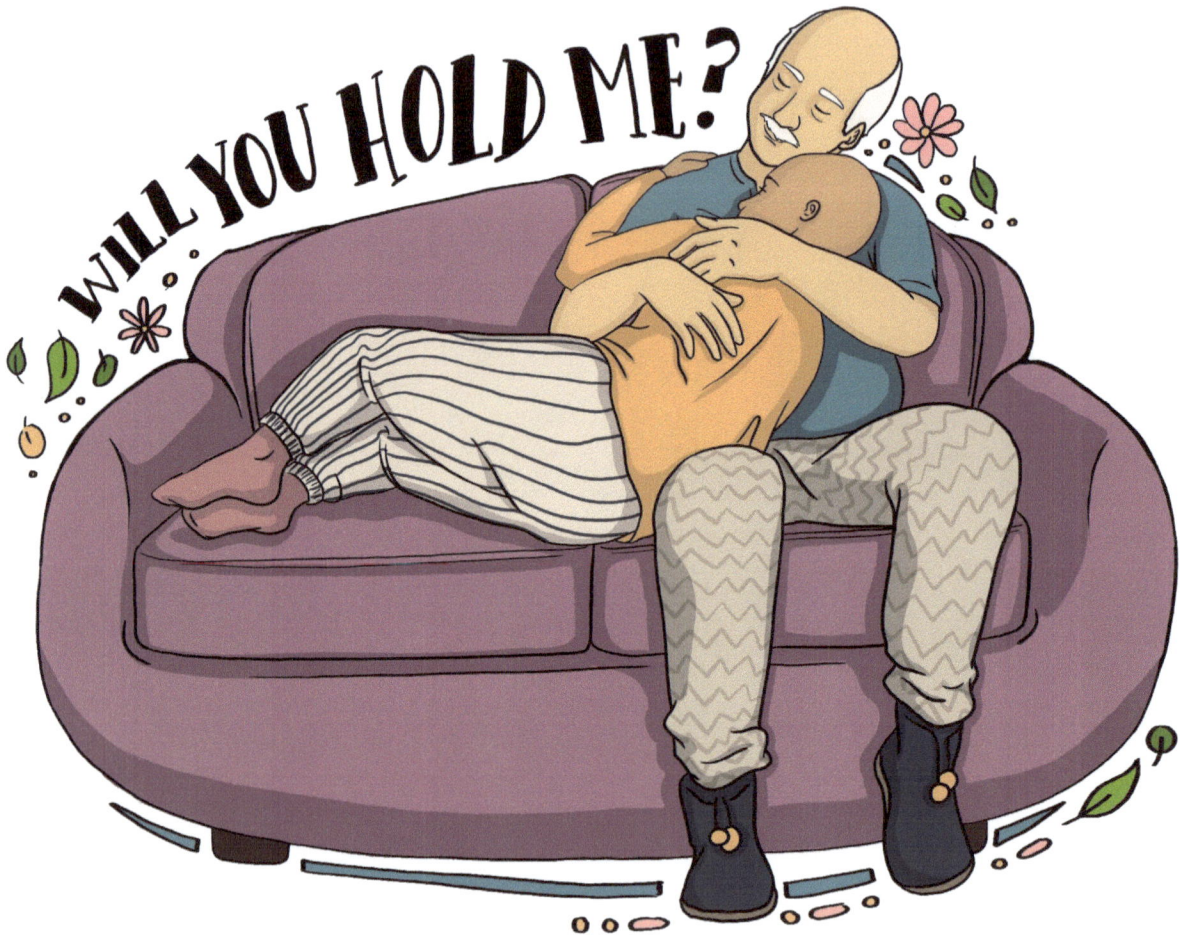

WILL YOU HOLD ME?

20

Sit down on the couch with your feet on the ground. Your partner sits next to you with their legs along the couch, perpendicular to your body. Then they place their head on your chest, allowing you to hold their upper body.

Pro-Tips

- This position allows a lot of relaxation for your partner, especially since they can listen to your heartbeat while being held.

- There is an extra sense of safety here, as they are being cradled with their upper body surrounded.

- Try holding your partner's upper arm, shoulder, neck, or back, or the side of their head. See what feels good to them.

- Another option is to squeeze your partner softly in time with their breathing. Hold tight while exhaling, and release on their inhale.

SAFE CRADLE

INTIMACY
●●●
LEVEL

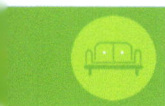

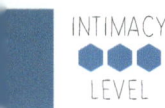

Sit upright with your legs spread to the sides, and invite your partner to sit in front of you, with their back to you. Your partner scoots back until they can lie down on their back and rest their head on your chest.

In this position of safety, your partner can caress your arms and legs, while you can caress them lovingly or hug them from behind.

Pro-Tips

- Be careful where you place your hands and arms; make sure your partner is comfortable with the locations you choose.

- To avoid arousal, place a pillow or a folded blanket between your pelvises.

- Try intertwining your legs (right with right, left with left).

- For extra security and calm, have your partner turn their head to one side to lie their face against your chest. You may then put your hand on their face or head to envelop them with caring touch.

- If both of you feel comfortable, place your hand on your partner's sternum (not the breasts, but just above them). You may also apply *slight* pressure as they breathe, if it feels good to them.

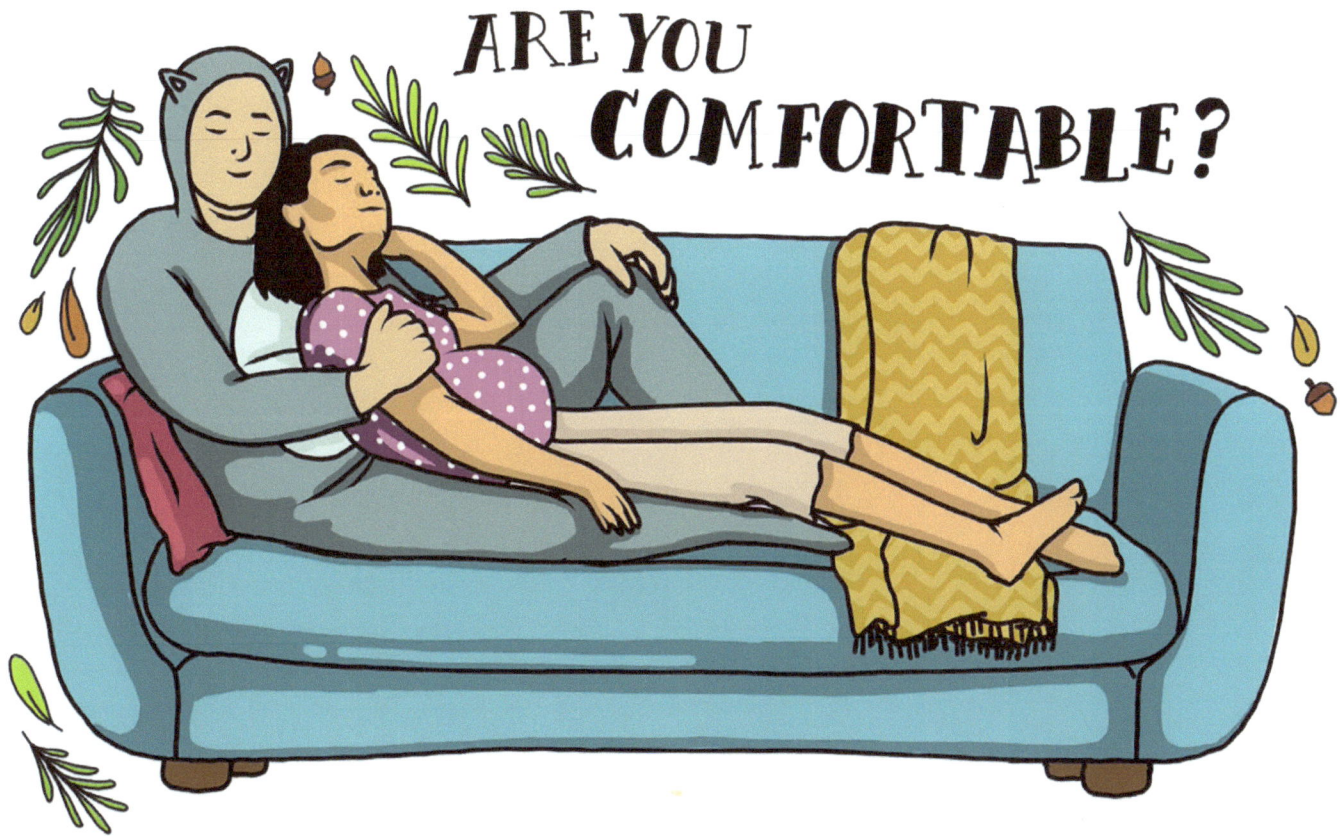

ARE YOU COMFORTABLE?

LYING DOWN SAFE CRADLE

This is a variation on the Safe Cradle where both people are lying down. You can try everything that relates to the Safe Cradle, just lying down. The bonus of this position is that your partner's back gets more of a stretch.

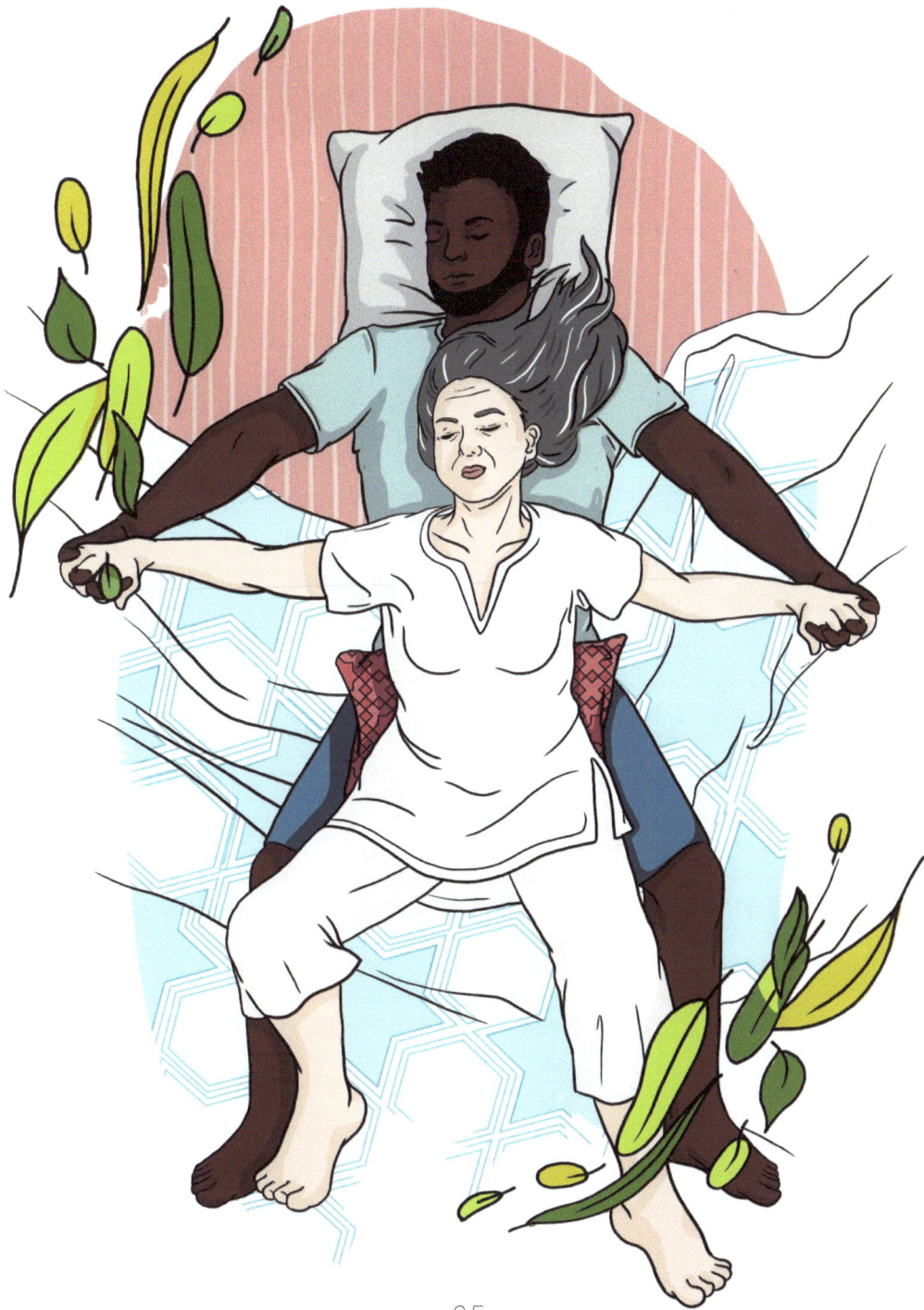

SLEEPING KID

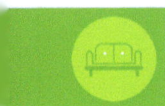

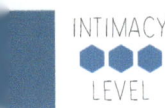

This position might be difficult to get into, but it's worth it. Sit on the couch with legs spread, so your partner can sit between your legs. They then shift to one side, perpendicular to your body, and bend their legs to go over yours. Now you can hug them with one arm under the crook of their knee and the other around their shoulders, bringing them in for a closer embrace.

This position is similar to "Listen to the Beat," only here your partner is seated between your legs.

Pro-Tips

- Allow your partner to come closer and rest their head on your chest.

- To increase intimacy, your hand can leave their shoulder and hold their head against your chest.

- Some people like to feel a gentle side-to-side rocking motion.

- This position allows your partner to curl up and be enveloped in a safe, loving, and caring bubble of security.

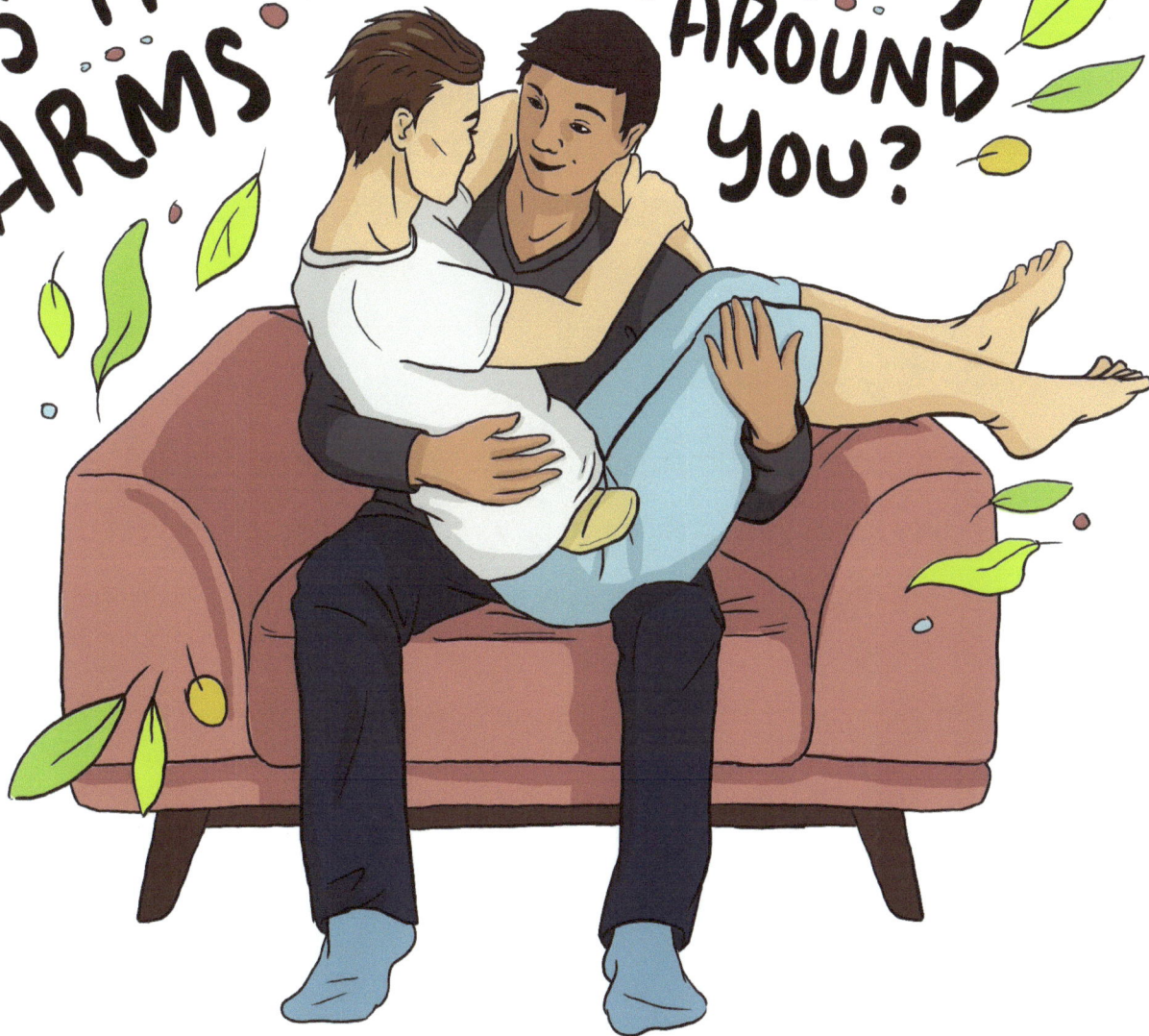

MIRROR IMAGE

As opposed to "Spooning," "Mirror Image" is when both people lie on their sides but face each other.

Just like in "Spooning," one of you lies on your bottom arm, while the other's bottom arm can rest under your neck, or stretch above their head or behind their own back.

Pro-Tips

- Playing "footsie" is another cute and fun way to interact.

- This is also a good opportunity to play with one another's hair.

- Your knees could intertwine or stay apart, or you can rest your knee on your partner's thigh.

- You can gaze at one another, but sometimes this can be too intense, so people choose to look elsewhere.

- Your top hands can touch and caress one another's top arm or body.

- You can dive into deeper intimacy levels by touching one another's faces.

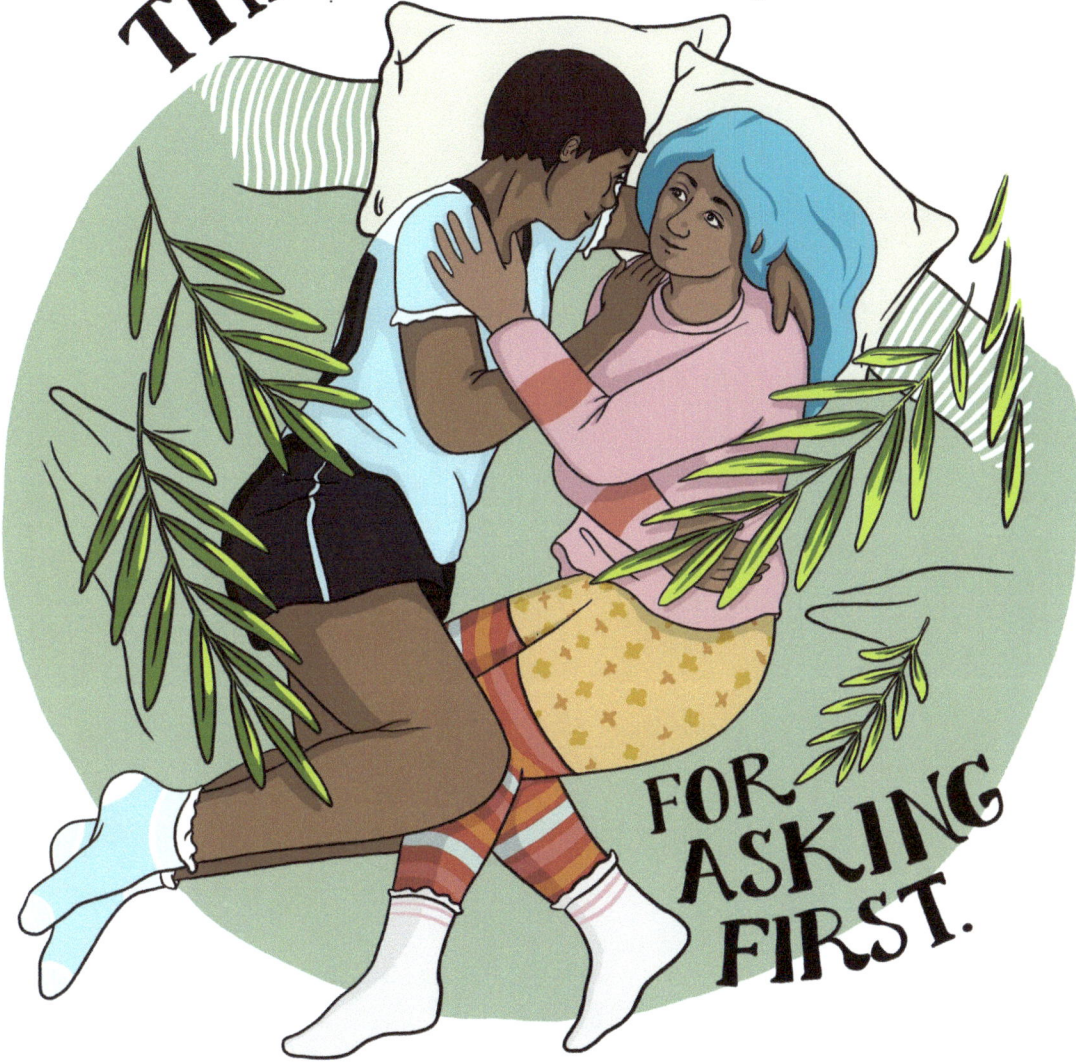

THANK YOU

FOR
ASKING
FIRST.

HUGS

SEATBELT HUG

The egalitarian hug. This hug is designed to have both parties "give and receive" the hug in the same way. When approaching for the hug, each of you tilts your head and upper body to the left (usually). That way, your head rests on your partner's right shoulder, with your right arm over and your left arm under.

Pro-Tips

- Approaching one another with your arms in the position of this hug will automatically signal to the other person how they can join the hug.

- You can decide on the intensity of the hug by how close your bodies get and for how long you hold the embrace.

- To really increase the intimacy of the hug, you can place your faces side by side or even cheek to cheek. Touching faces together is a very intimate experience.

- Try this hug with your heads on the right side instead of the left, with arms switched. Some people like this variation because it puts both partners' hearts close together.

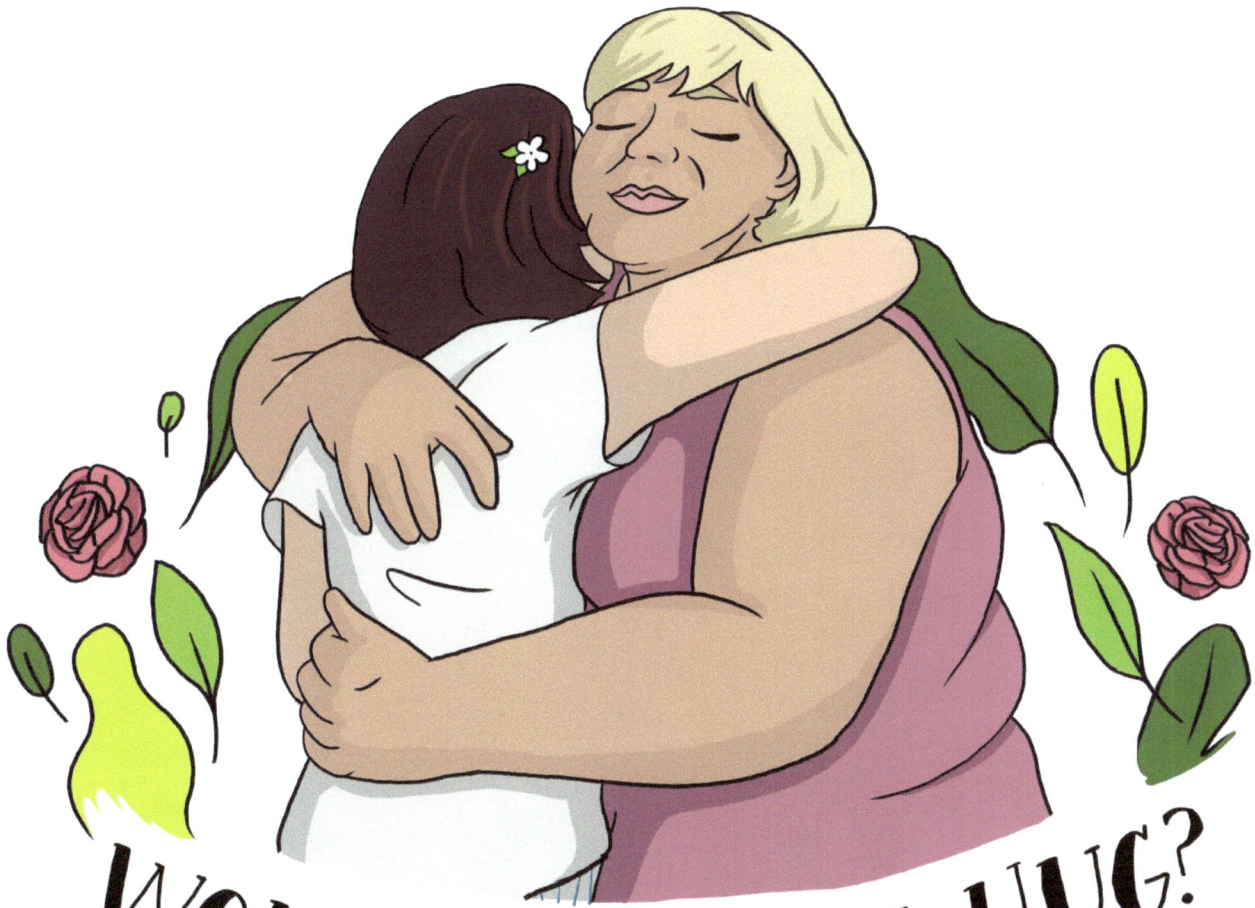

WOULD YOU LIKE A HUG?

ENVELOPE HUG

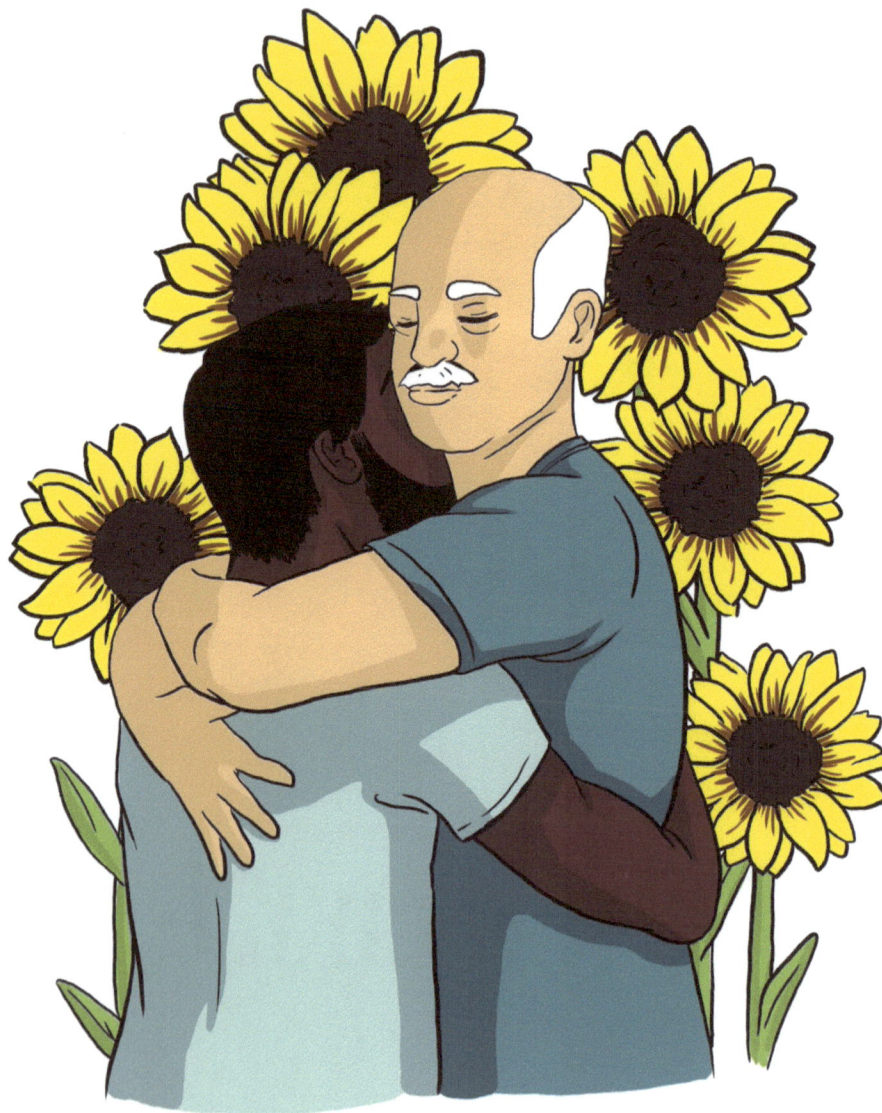

34

This hug is useful when there's a significant height difference between the huggers. The taller person positions their arms above their partner's shoulders or arms, enveloping their whole upper body.

Pro-Tips

- If the height difference is substantial, the shorter person can ask to rest their head on the other's upper chest.

- In order to achieve higher levels of relaxation, take a deep breath together. As you exhale, try relaxing your whole upper bodies and sink into the hug together. This changes the whole hugging experience.

- Shorter people tend to go up on their toes to give hugs. If you're the taller partner, you can walk a little closer to signal to the other person that they don't need to stay on their toes and can relax. Another option is to take a wide stance, to lower your torso without bending over.

BLANKET HUG

This hug is like a warm blanket of care and one-way attention. Stand behind your partner and ask to place your hands around them. This allows them to completely give in to your touch.

Pro-Tips

- The person in front can rest their head on your shoulder.

- You can lean on one another for support and a feeling of weight.

- The hand positions you use while standing behind your partner can create different levels of intimacy. You can try it with:
  - Both hands under your partner's arms and hanging on their shoulders (like the shoulder straps of a backpack).
  - One hand on the upper chest.
  - One hand on the stomach.
  - Your arms on the side of their body.
  - Any combination of these.

- Putting your heads close to one another and touching cheeks may feel very intimate.

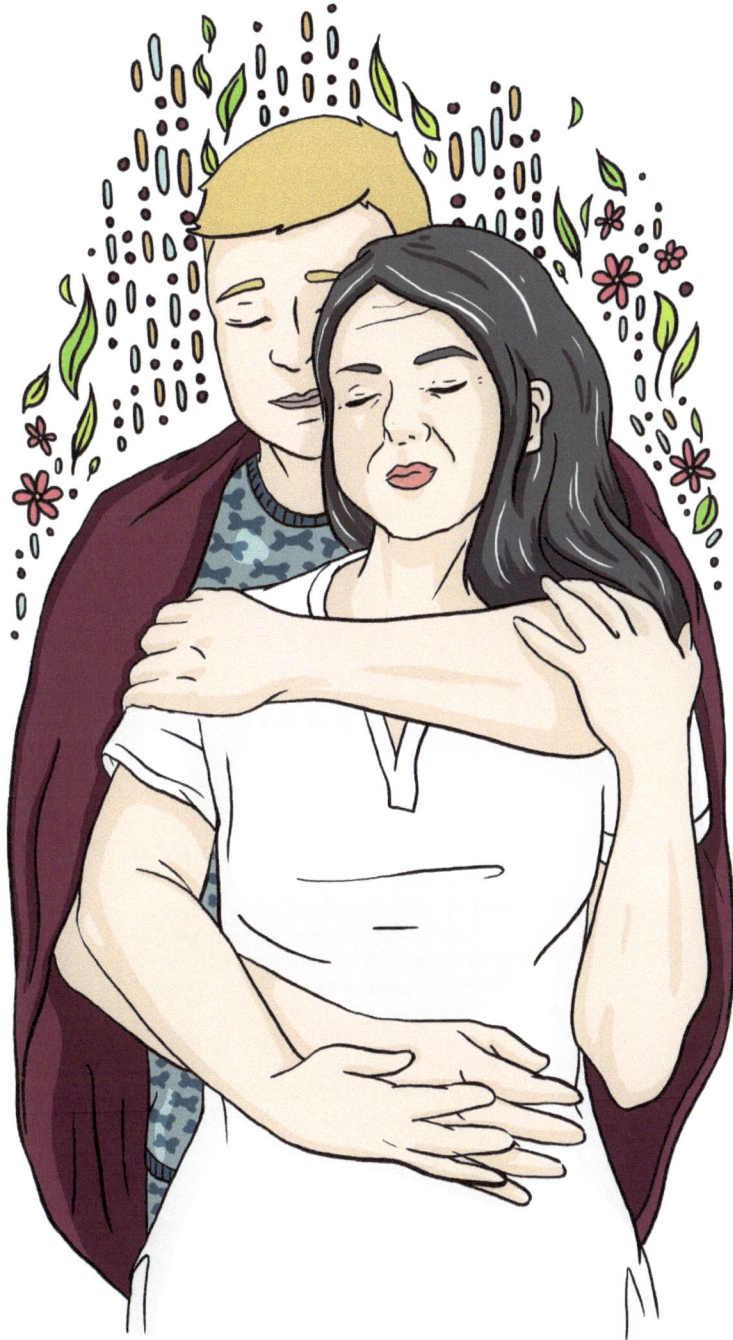

GROUP CUDDLES

HAND LOOP

This is a good position to ease people into feeling more comfortable with touch in a group setting. Everyone sits cross-legged in a circle, facing in, and holds hands. Each person massages the hand on their right, while their left hand gets a massage from the person on their left. The only contact is hands, and people are sitting and looking at one another but not necessarily at the people on their sides, which can facilitate conversation.

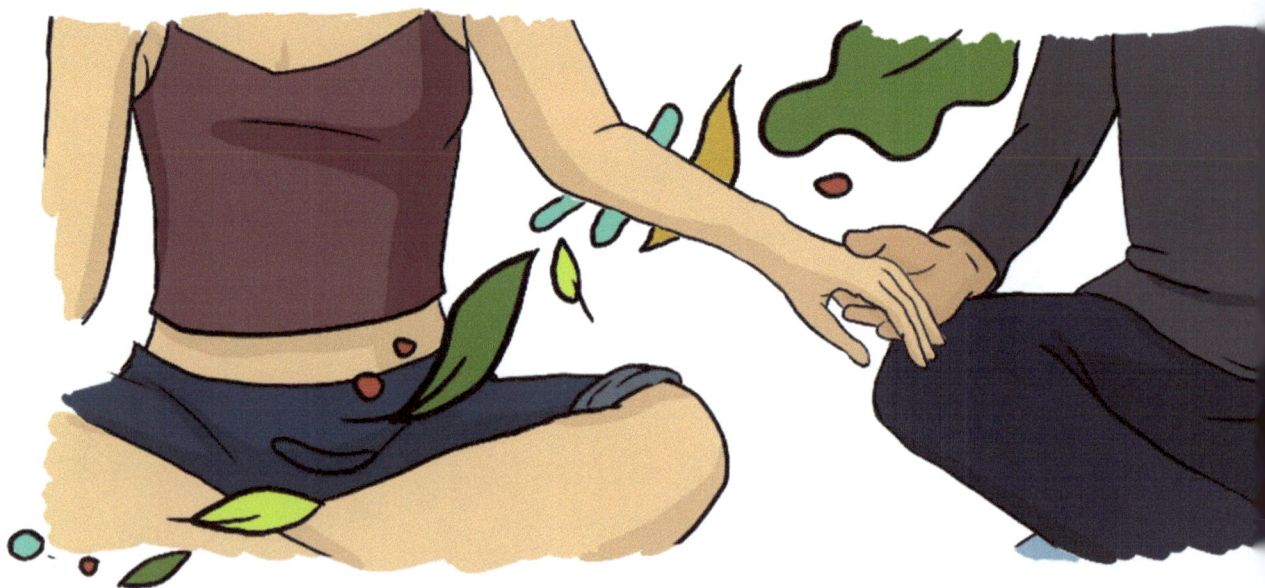

Pro-Tips

- It might take a moment to get used to massaging someone's hand using only one hand, but it gets easier.

- If the person on the right wants you to, you can move from the hand up to the wrist and the forearm.

- After a while, you can switch directions.

- You can also completely change places, Mad Hatter tea-party style.

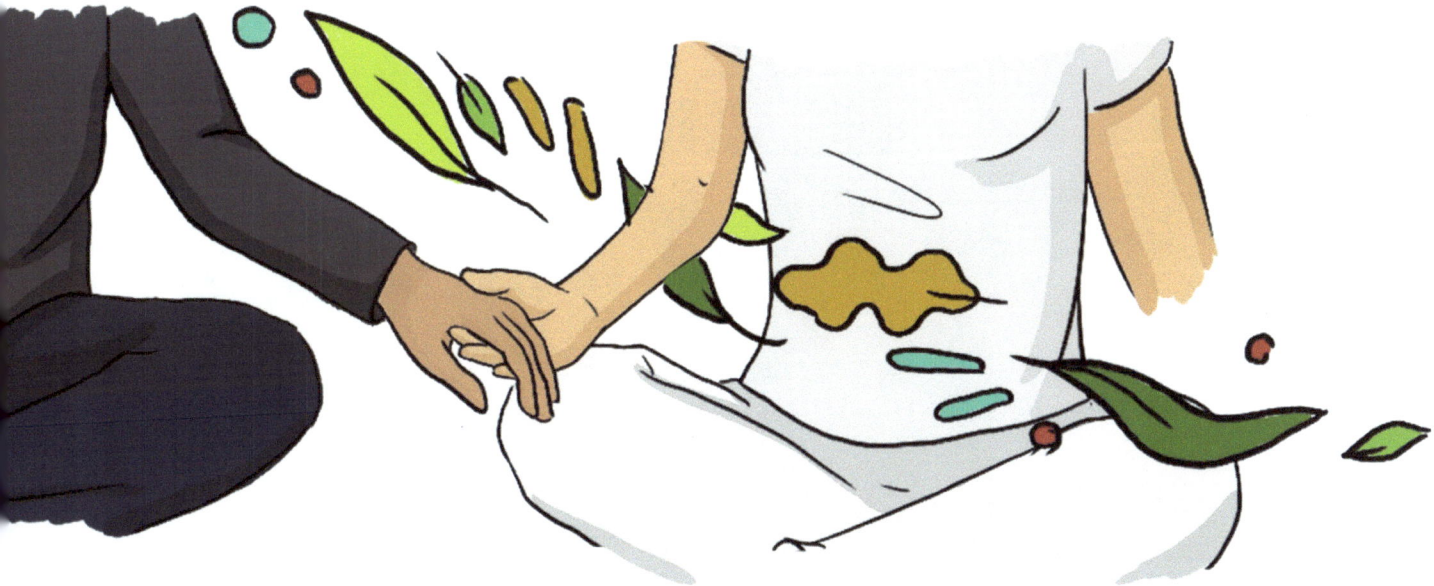

MASSAGE TRAIN

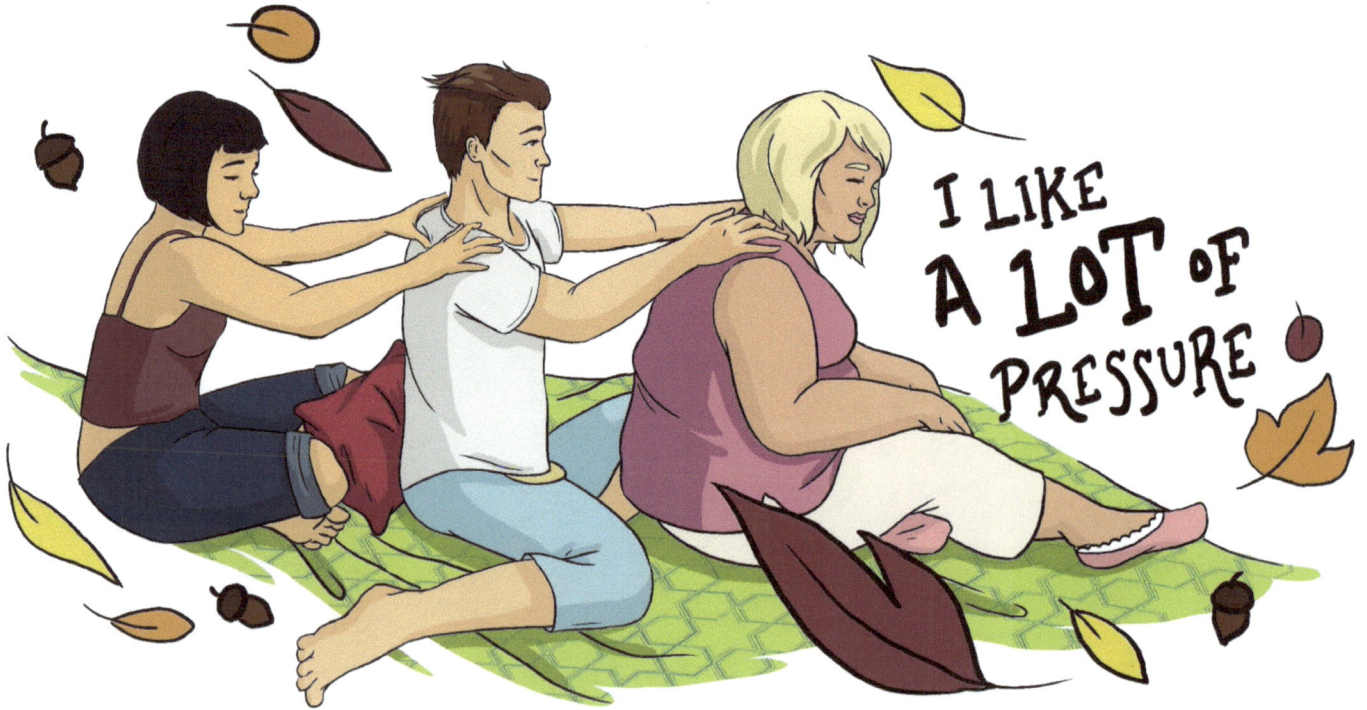

I LIKE A LOT OF PRESSURE

Reciprocity at its best. Form a line of people sitting one behind the other, facing in the same direction. Each person will communicate with and massage the person in front of them, while being asked and massaged by the person behind them.

Pro-Tips

- Don't forget to turn around, so that the people at the ends get their share.
- Another option is to close the line into a circle.
- Depending on space, you can make two or more rows.

SPOON DRAWER

A spoon drawer is when more than two people cuddle in the "Spooning" position. This can be done by adding more people to either side.
This position creates a combination of giving and receiving. At times, people might get confused between whose hands are whose.

Pro-Tips

- The smallest spoon in the "drawer" may choose to change their position and lie on their back (like in "Gonna Be OK") or face the rest of the spoons (like in "Mirror Image").

- You may want to place your arm underneath the neck of the person in front of you. This usually also leads to your hand touching the person in front of them, which gives an opportunity to play with their hair or put your hand under their neck as well.

- You will touch and be touched by more than one person in this position; please make sure everyone consents to each type of touch.

- Try having everyone synchronize their breath.

- Another interesting sensation is to have everyone take a deep breath and hum in a low tone on the exhale.

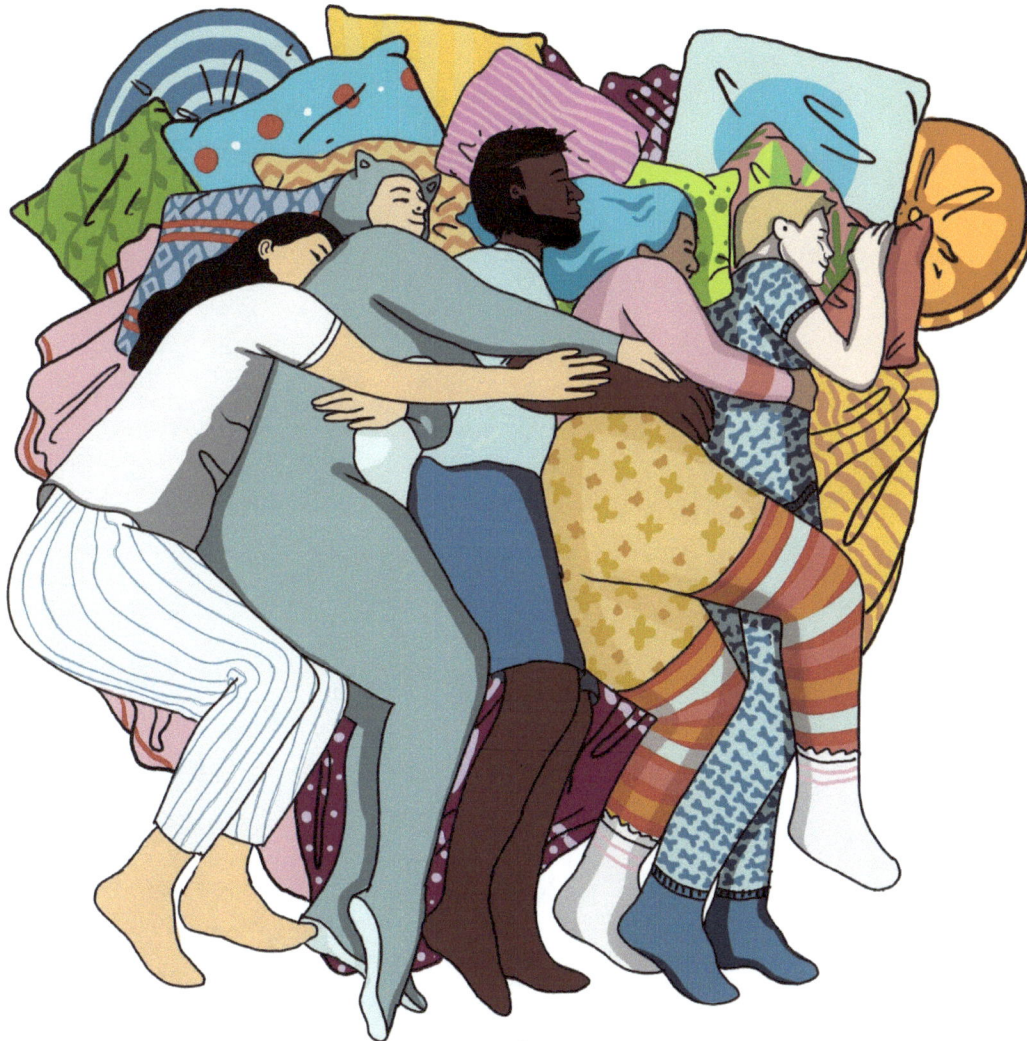

LAUGH CIRCLE

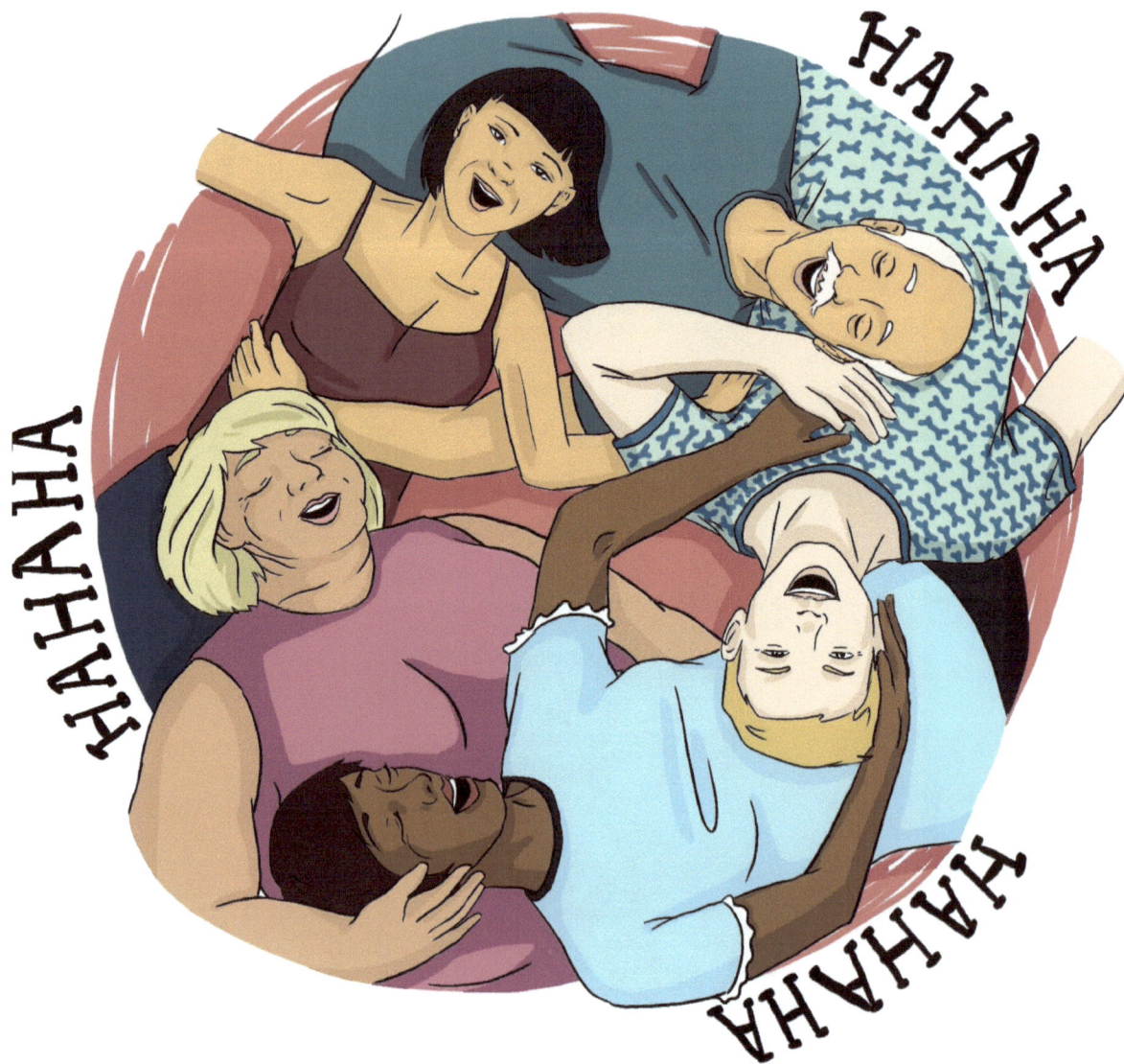

This is a fun one! Have people lie down on the floor and form a circle, so that each person's head is resting on the next person's stomach, all the way around, until everyone's head is on someone else's stomach. Then at some point, someone starts to laugh, which will make their tummy move. That will cause the head of the person lying on them to bounce, which will likely make *them* laugh and bounce the next person—until everyone is giggling uncontrollably.

Pro-Tips

- If people don't start to laugh, don't be discouraged—it doesn't work every time!

  Even without laughter, it is still a good position to take care of one another while receiving touch.

- The angle of people's positions will change according to the number of people in the circle, so you might have to shift every time someone joins or leaves the circle.

- Try laughing while resting your heads in other locations, positions, and angles.

PUPPY PILE

Kinda what it sounds like: just a big, warm pile of everyone. Have a few people lie on their backs or stomachs next to one another (or with their feet next to one another's heads). Then have people start joining on top of them, either perpendicular to everyone or straight on top.

It is very important that everyone joins slowly and carefully. There are more body parts involved than we're normally used to, so make sure that everyone is comfortable and no one is being squished or poked.

As with all group cuddles, if someone wants to join the group, it is important to ask everyone in the group whether they are okay with that person joining, even if they don't expect to be touching. You never know how things might move and change.

Pro-Tips

- Be careful about stomachs, faces, and genitals. These are sensitive areas that might get hurt by a stray elbow or too much weight, so watch out!

- The people on top should watch their elbows, knees, and anything that has a small surface area. Applying weight on a small area could hurt others. Please shift slowly.

- Another thing to think about is how arms and legs bend. Make sure that everyone is comfortable and no appendage is being pressured in the wrong direction.

- Feeling the pressure of another body on yours can feel good, but please pay attention to everyone in the pile and make sure everyone is constantly okay.

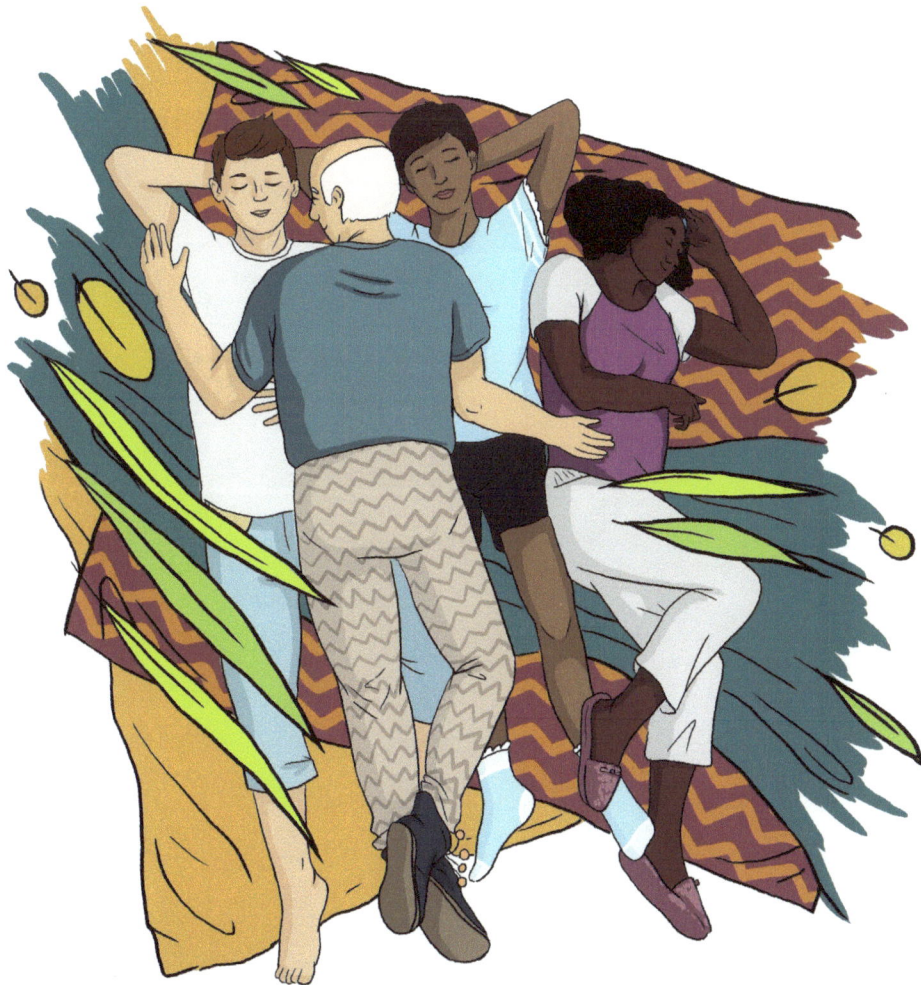

CUDDLE-CULE

"Cuddle-cule" is a mashup of "cuddle" and "molecule." It's a general term for any combination of people cuddling with one another, but not necessarily all connected directly.

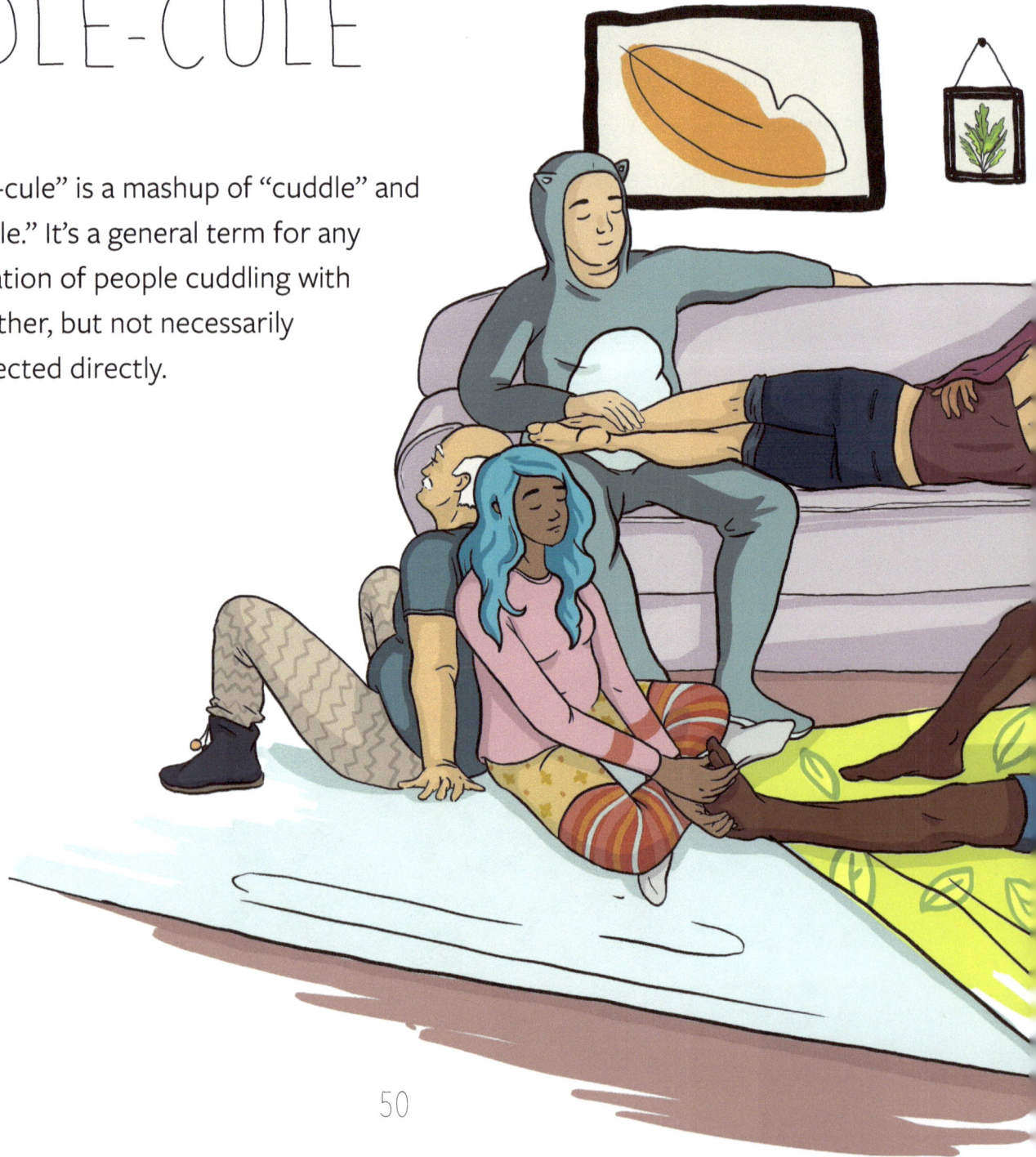

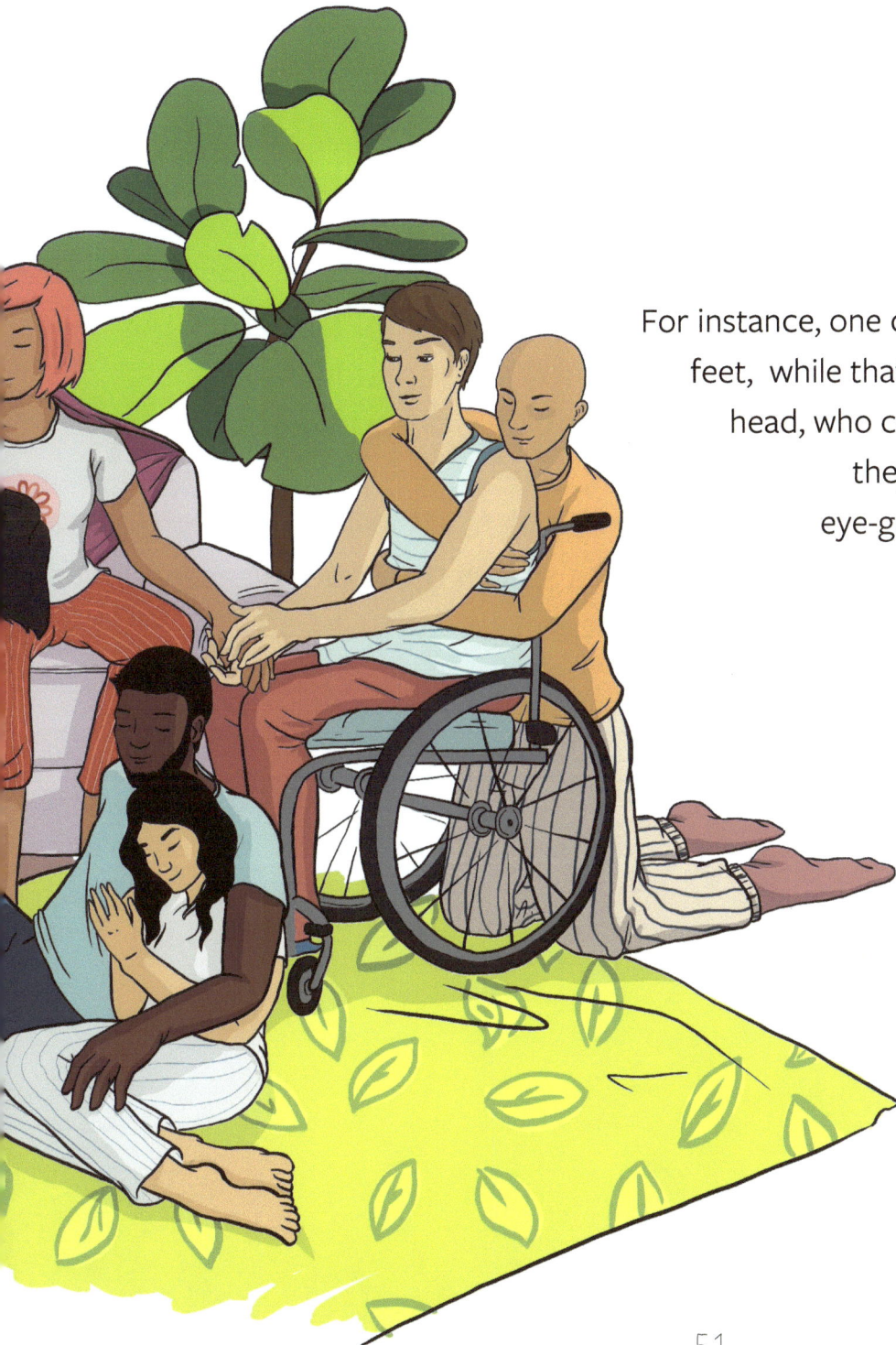

For instance, one could be massaging another's feet, while that person rubs someone else's head, who caresses another's arms, while they spoon with someone who's eye-gazing with another, and so on and so on...

EPILOGUE

We hope you've enjoyed exploring new horizons in your cuddling. Even the most experienced cuddler is always on a journey of learning, experiencing, and bettering themselves.

If you'd like to learn more about the book and stay in the know, please visit www.thebookofcuddles.com and join our list.

May safe touch and intentional attention bring joy and health into your lives,

Yoni and Cecilia

ACKNOWLEDGEMENTS

Soleiman Bolour

Leela Sinha

Janet Trevino, M.A.

Michelle Renee

Keeley Shoup

Sundria Sam

Anna Smidebush

Jennifer Guise Rahner

Adora Diana

Allison Edenzon

Jessy Mijnssen

Melissa Kelly

Justin L.

Sarah Belzile

Sarah Grey (GreyEditing.com)
    for copyediting

A personal thank to Madelon Guinazzo and Adam Lippin for creating Cuddlist.com, and to Marcia Baczynski and Reid Mihalko for creating CuddleParty.com.

Yoni: I'd like to especially thank my parents for giving me all the cuddles growing up, and Alexis for her unwavering support in all my endeavors.

Cecilia: Thank you to my parents, siblings and friends for their love and acceptance of all the off-beat ways I choose to express myself.

Find out more about the book:

www.TheBookofCuddles.com

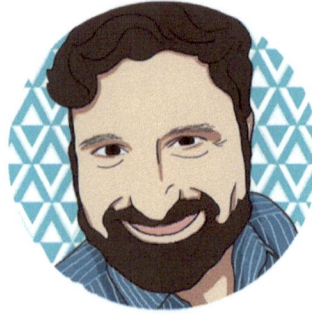

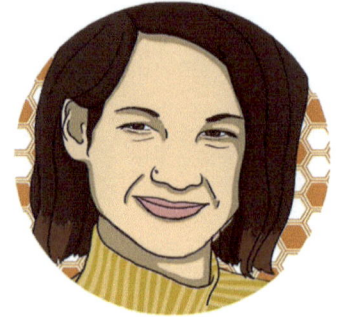

Find out more about the author Yoni:

Yoni Alkan is a San Francisco–based sexual educator and consultant with a doctorate in human sexuality. He is also a Cuddle Party facilitator with CuddleParty.com and a one-on-one cuddler with Cuddlist.com.
Learn more about his work at www.yonialkan.com and at www.elementsofsexuality.com.

Find out more about the illustrator Cecilia:

Cecilia Li is a Cleveland-based artist and animator. She is a certified cuddling professional through both Cuddlist and Cuddle Party.
You can find examples of her artwork at www.cxlmotion.com or keep up to date on her cuddling events and various other projects at www.cuddlewithc.com.

www.ingramcontent.com/pod-product-compliance
Lightning Source LLC
Chambersburg PA
CBHW060820270326
41930CB00003B/102